Bending Adversity: The Story of My Struggle Against Scoliosis

Bending Adversity: The Story of My Struggle Against Scoliosis

Éric Braza Torres

To my family, friends, professionals, and all the people who accompany me in this process, and especially to those who have gone through, are going through, or will go through the same as me.

The Purpose Of The Book

The purpose of this book is to share my personal story of battling scoliosis, with the aim of inspiring and providing hope to those facing similar challenges. Through my experience, I hope to offer an honest and sincere insight into the physical, emotional, and mental hurdles I encountered during my treatment.

Furthermore, this book also seeks to raise awareness about scoliosis and its impact on the everyday lives of those affected by it. By sharing my story, I hope to help educate and raise awareness within society about this medical condition.

Lastly, this book also serves the purpose of expressing gratitude to all the people who have supported me throughout my recovery process, as well as shedding light on what all scoliosis patients go through. I want to demonstrate that with determination, perseverance, and the right support, it is possible to overcome the challenges that scoliosis may present and achieve a fulfilling and satisfying life.

0 – Who I am?

Before I begin telling my story, it's important for you to know who I am. I am Éric, Éric Braza, and I am fourteen years old at the time of writing this, currently in my third year of high school (ESO) in a school in Catalonia. I consider myself a good student, jovial, and optimistic… and I am a person who has been living with scoliosis for a few years now. Not only that, but I have had to deal with wearing a corset and frequent visits to the doctor for adjustments. But I have also had moments of overcoming and learning through my experience with this condition.

Currently, I find myself in a challenging situation regarding my condition. I am in growth phase 5 out of a total of 6, and I am wearing a brace. This means that when I reach the end of phase 6, my orthopedic specialist, my parents, and I will have to say if a surgery is necessary or not to correct the condition.

With that said, I think there's nothing more interesting to tell about myself, so I invite you to keep reading to get a sense of the situation and begin to understand my story and how I have reached the point where I am right now.

1- The Diagnostic

Honestly, I don't remember the exact day when my life changed forever. I was really young, probably I had four or five years old. At that time, I didn't have any pain or anything like that, but I went to the doctor for my regular annual check-up. Upon arriving at the clinic and after a series of routine tests and examinations, I received the news that I had unspecified kyphosis in the thoracic area. Although, the pediatrician didn't give it much importance and mentioned it like it hadn't importance.

At that moment, they explained to my mother that kyphosis is a condition that affects the vertebrae in the thoracic (upper) region of the back. Being quite young, I don't remember that, but my parents did worry, although not excessively (since at that time it didn't seem to influence me in any way).

A few days later, due to the news of my condition, my mother enrolled me in various extracurricular activities that I honestly hated. Among these activities were dance and swimming, because they wanted my spine to grow straight and strong. In addition to participating in these activities a couple of times a week, my parents constantly tried to correct my posture to counteract the problem. "sit down straight," "sit properly," "mind your back…

THE DETECTION

Scoliosis is a medical condition that can be difficult to detect, especially in its early stages. In my case, the process of diagnosing scoliosis was a bit lengthy. In fact, several years passed from that initial diagnosis of kyphosis to the diagnostic. During those years, everything seemed normal, but it eventually led to receiving the appropriate treatment for my condition.

As I mentioned, the years went by, and we were in the midst of a lockdown, which meant staying at home all the time. As a result, I would spend long periods of time sitting. During that time, I used tp play video games for long times, and I couldn't participate in dance or swimming. On top of that, I was in the fastest stage of my growth: pre-adolescence. I remember that my back started to hurt frequently, and my parents noticed that there was a visible deviation in my spine. Due to the lockdown, it was impossible to schedule a non-urgent medical visit, but as soon as it was possible to request an appointment, my mother did so.

First, I went to the pediatrician with my father, and he explained my situation and the worry about the pain, as well as the sudden visible curvature that had appeared on my back. My father also requested X-rays to examine my spine. Finally, I was referred to a specialist. After a couple of months more or less, we were called to have the X-rays done and proceed with a visit to the local hospital to discuss the results.

The process of getting the X-rays done was relatively quick, but also uncomfortable. I was asked to remove my shirt and stand in front of a large machine while a technician took X-rays of my spine. They assured me that the procedure wouldn't cause any pain, but I was still a bit nervous.

After the X-rays were taken, my father and I went to the orthopedic specialist's office. The specialist informed us that they had detected an abnormal curvature in my spine and that I needed to have a visit at another hospital. The curvature was significant enough to require some orthopedic device.

It was at that moment when we realized that my back pain was not just a temporary discomfort, it was a symptom of a much larger problem. The curvature in my spine was diagnosed as idiopathic scoliosis.

From there, the process of treating my scoliosis began. This process involved several visits to the orthopedic specialist at the other hospital in my area. There, I received additional tests and examinations. Finally, at the age of twelve, my orthopedic specialist made the decision to start using a corset to try to treat the condition.

I have to say that wearing the corset was completely voluntary, and no one forced me to do it. However, my parents and I made the decision to use it because we wanted to avoid surgery at all costs due to the potential side effects and the tedious recovery process it would involve.

Looking back, I'm grateful that they found my scoliosis in time and that I can get the right treatment to try to prevent the curve from getting worse. If my mom hadn't insisted on taking me to the doctor because of my back pain, it's possible that they would have discovered my scoliosis later, and it would have been harder to treat.

In summary, the detection of scoliosis can be a lengthy and tedious process, but it is crucial to ensure that the appropriate treatment is received early. If you experience persistent back pain or have a family history of scoliosis, make sure to talk to your parents about scheduling a medical appointment.

THE MEDICAL TESTS

When I was diagnosed with scoliosis at the age of 12, I had to go through several medical tests to confirm the diagnosis and see the severity of the curve in my spine. These tests were important for the doctors to create a suitable treatment plan for my condition.

The first test I had to evaluate my scoliosis was X-rays. The process of taking X-rays was a bit scary for me, but the radiology technicians were kind and patient. The X-rays allowed the doctors to see the curve in my spine and assess its severity. They could determine from the X-rays that the curve in my spine was significant enough to justify a more extensive treatment plan.

After the X-rays, I underwent a series of physical exams to evaluate my mobility and strength in the upper part of my body. The doctor also asked me to walk and observed me from different angles to evaluate my posture and how I moved.

Another important test I had was a flexibility test. I was asked to bend forward and touch my toes. Through this test, the doctors could evaluate the flexibility of my spine and determine how flexible it was.

Although these tests were necessary to evaluate my scoliosis and determine the best class of treatment, they can also be a bit tedious to receive. However, the doctors and radiology technicians who attended to me were kind and patient, and they explained the whole process to me clearly. They also allowed me to ask questions and calmed me throughout the process.

THE IMPACT OF THE DIAGNOSTIC IN MY LIVE

When I was diagnosed with scoliosis at the age of twelve, I didn't fully understand the impact this condition would have on my life until later. While I knew I had a curvature in my spine, I had no idea how it would affect my day-to-day life and my future.

At first, I thought scoliosis was just a physical condition and that it wouldn't have any other impact on my life. However, I soon realized that scoliosis could impact much more than just my posture and my ability to do certain physical activities, especially as I was starting adolescence.

One of the first impacts the diagnosis had on my life was the fact that I had to start wearing a corset to treat my scoliosis at the age of twelve. The corset was uncomfortable and restrictive, and it was a big adjustment for my daily life. I had to learn how to move and do activities while wearing it, which was often uncomfortable and required a lot of effort.

Furthermore, having to wear that made me feel different from my friends and classmates. I was frequently asked what that strange object I was wearing was, and I had to explain my condition to them. Although my friends were understanding, I sometimes felt a bit excluded and different.

The diagnosis of scoliosis had several impacts on my life. One of them was the need to make lifestyle adjustments to ensure that my condition didn't get worse. This included avoiding some sports and activities and engaging in others that could help prevent the progression of scoliosis. For instance, I took up swimming again, even though I used to dislike it, and made sure to maintain good posture at all times.

I also had to do specific physical therapy exercises to make my back stronger, which required time and effort. Sometimes, I felt frustrated because it seemed like I had to put in more work than my friends to maintain my physical health and well-being.

The diagnosis of scoliosis also had an impact on my emotional well-being. I was sometimes feeling sad or anxious about dealing with a chronic condition and having to wear a corset. I also worried about how it would affect my future and my ability to do certain things.

However, over time, I learned to accept my condition and find ways to adapt and overcome the challenges that scoliosis presented. I learned to appreciate the importance of small things and not worry about things I couldn't change.

I also found support from others who had similar experiences, such as other kids and teenagers with scoliosis. Through social media and different forums, I connected with them, which helped me feel that I wasn't alone and that there were others who understood what I was going through. It made me appreciate my own situation and realize that there were much more severe circumstances or other people who were having a really hard time.

In conclusion, the diagnosis of scoliosis had a significant impact on my life. I had to make lifestyle adjustments and face physical and emotional challenges, but I also learned to accept my condition and find ways to adapt and overcome the obstacles that the condition developed.

2- The Curve

In the previous chapter, we discussed the process of detection and diagnosis of scoliosis. In this chapter, I will focus on the topic of the curve.

The curvature of the spine is the characteristic feature of scoliosis and what sets it apart from other spinal conditions.

In this chapter, we will delve into understanding what scoliosis is from an anatomical and physiological perspective. We will explore the different types of scoliosis and how they can be identified, all explained in a way that is accessible to everyone. I will share my knowledge and experience, based on what I have learned from specialists' explanations and my own curiosity about the subject.

Additionally, we will discuss how the curve affects overall health and the risks and complications associated with scoliosis. It is important to understand the severity of the situation and how it can impact a person's quality of life.

WHAT IS SCOLIOISIS

Scoliosis is a medical condition characterized by an abnormal curvature of the spine. This curvature can occur anywhere along the spine, but it is typically seen in the thoracic or lumbar region.

The curve can take the shape of an "S."

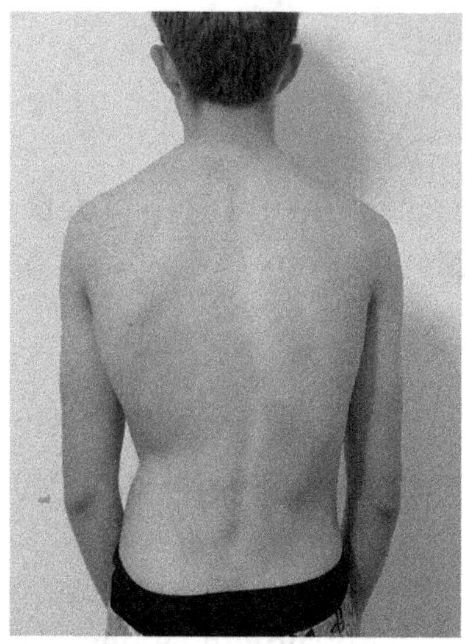

(my case)

In addition, it can be in the shape of a "C" and can range from mild to severe, depending on the degree of curvature.

Most people have a slight curvature in the spine, known as a physiological curve. However, in scoliosis, the curve is significantly bigger, which can cause imbalances in the body and health problems. The curve can affect both physical appearance and body normal function.

There are several types of scoliosis, including idiopathic, congenital, neuromuscular, and degenerative. Idiopathic scoliosis is the most common form, and its exact cause is unknown. It is believed to be hereditary and primarily affects children and adolescents during their growth period. I should mention that my scoliosis, like most cases, is idiopathic, although my parents are not aware of any family members who have had the condition.

In congenital scoliosis, the spine develops abnormally in the uterus. This can be caused by various factors, including genetic problems, exposure to toxic substances, infections during pregnancy, and other factors.

Neuromuscular scoliosis occurs as a result of a neurological or muscular disease, such as cerebral disfunction or muscular dystrophy.

Degenerative scoliosis is a condition that occurs as a result of natural wear and developing of the spine.

The degree of curvature is measured using a method called the Cobb angle. This method measures the angle between the upper and lower vertebrae in the curve. If the Cobb angle is less than 10 degrees, it is considered a normal curvature. If the angle is 10 to 25 degrees, it is considered mild scoliosis. If the angle is 25 to 40 degrees, it is considered moderate, and if it exceeds 40 degrees, it is considered severe.

Personally, when I was diagnosed, I had a 36-degree curvature, which was considered moderate scoliosis. If the angle had been over 40 degrees, it would have been considered severe scoliosis, while if it had been less than 30 degrees, it would have been considered soft.

The curvature of the spine can affect the body's function in various ways. It can modify posture and balance, leading to coordination problems and falls. The curve can also affect lung capacity and the heart, increasing the probability of respiratory difficulties and heart problems in the future.

In conclusion, scoliosis is a common medical condition characterized by an abnormal curvature of the spine. It can affect both physical appearance and bodily function. There are various types of scoliosis, and the degree of curvature is measured using the Cobb angle. It is important for patients with scoliosis to be evaluated by a doctor and receive appropriate treatment to prevent complications and improve their quality of life.

TYPES OF SCOLIOSIS

As mentioned briefly in the previous chapter, scoliosis can be classified into three main types based on the shape of the curve: C-shaped scoliosis, S-shaped scoliosis, and double S-shaped scoliosis. C-shaped scoliosis is the most common form of scoliosis and is characterized by a curve shaped like the letter "C" in the spine. S-shaped scoliosis has an S-shaped curve in the spine, while double S-shaped scoliosis has two S-shaped curves.

C-shaped scoliosis can be caused by various factors, including muscle imbalances, hip misalignment, and growth issues, among others. In most cases, C-shaped scoliosis is soft and does not require treatment. However, in severe cases, a corset may be necessary or, in extreme cases, surgery.

S-shaped scoliosis is less common than C-shaped scoliosis and is characterized by an S-shaped curve in the spine. S-shaped scoliosis can be caused by many things, like the other types of scoliosis. Like C-shaped scoliosis, in most cases, S-shaped scoliosis soft, although treating these cases can be slightly more challenging due to the double curve in the back.

HOW SCOLIOSIS IMPACTS HEALTH

Here are the main risks and complications associated with scoliosis:

Back pain:
Scoliosis can cause back pain, especially in the lumbar region. The abnormal curvature of the spine can put pressure on the nerves and muscles of the back, leading to pain and stiffness.

Respiratory problems:
In severe cases, scoliosis can affect the lungs' capacity to function properly. The abnormal curvature of the spine can compress the lungs and make breathing more difficult. This can result in fatigue, shortness of breath, and other respiratory problems.

Cardiac issues:
Scoliosis can also impact heart health. If the spinal curve is severe, it can compress the chest cavity and impact the heart's ability to pump blood effectively. This can increase the risk of cardiovascular issues such as high blood pressure and heart failure.

Digestive problems:
Scoliosis can modify the digestive system as well. The abnormal curvature of the spine can compress the stomach and intestines, leading to digestive issues such as acid reflux, constipation, and diarrhea.

Sleep disturbances:
Scoliosis can also impact sleep quality. The abnormal curvature of the spine can make it difficult to find a comfortable sleeping position, resulting in insomnia and other sleep-related problems.

Emotional issues:
Scoliosis can have an impact on a person's mental and emotional well-being. The condition can affect self-pride and self-confidence, particularly in children and adolescents.

In conclusion, scoliosis is a complex condition that can have various effects on the body and overall health. Proper management and treatment, including medical interventions and emotional support, are crucial in minimizing the risks and complications associated with scoliosis.

MY CASE

Fortunately, I have only experienced a few mild symptoms of the condition. The most significant issue I personally faced was back pain. Back pain is common in older individuals, but not as common in teenagers like myself.

I had moderate back pain, mainly in my neck and left trapezius muscle. This pain was caused by the development of significant muscle tension in the upper back due to my scoliosis. As for other conditions, I have not experienced any that supposed a challenge in my daily life, so I can't complain too much.

3- The Desicion

Choosing the appropriate treatment for my scoliosis was one of the most important decisions we had to make on the journey towards correction. There were different options available, ranging from physical therapy and occupational therapy to surgery and wearing a brace. In this chapter, I will explore how we made the decision to use a brace to treat my scoliosis and how it impacted both my family and me. I will also discuss the different treatment options we researched and why we ultimately decided that a brace was the best choice for me. This chapter will also focus on my family's reaction to the decision and how we navigated the process together.

TREATMENT OPTIONS

Scoliosis is a medical condition that can be treated in various ways. The treatment will depend on several factors, including the patient's age, the severity of the bend of the spinal curvature, and the cause of the scoliosis. In this chapter, I will attempt to showcase the different treatment options available to correct scoliosis.

Observation and Monitoring

In mild cases of scoliosis, regular observation and monitoring are often recommended to track the progression of the curve. This may involve regular visits to the doctor for X-rays and spinal measurements. If the curvature does not get worse, the patient may not need any further treatment. Activities such as dancing or swimming are frequently recommended in these cases.

Physical Therapy

Physical therapy can help strengthen the muscles and improve the posture of patients with scoliosis. Specific exercises can help alleviate pain and prevent further spinal curvature. Additionally, physical therapy can also help improve flexibility and mobility. (My physical therapist combined this option with the corset and monitoring.)

Chiropractic Care

Chiropractic care is another treatment option that some individuals with scoliosis may consider. Chiropractors work to correct spinal alignment through manual adjustments. While chiropractic care may provide some pain relief, more research is needed to determine its effectiveness as a treatment for scoliosis.

Corset

Corsets are devices used to treat scoliosis in children and adolescents whose bones are still growing. It works by exerting constant pressure on the spine, which helps reduce the progression of the curve. There are different types of corset available, such as the Milwaukee corset (my second one) and the Boston corset (my first one), among others. The doctor or physical therapist will determine which is most suitable for the patient based on the location and severity of the curve.

FIRST CORSET

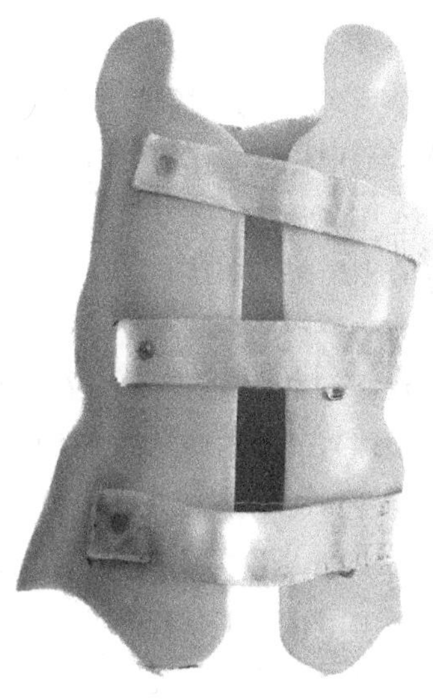

SECOND CORSET (ACTUAL ONE)

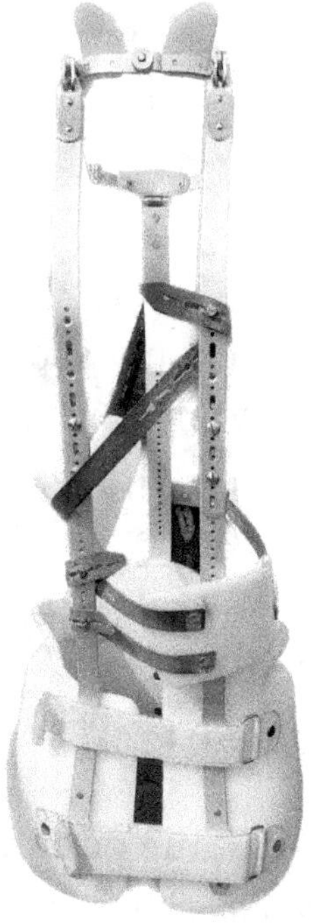

Surgery
Surgery is a more aggressive treatment option for scoliosis and is generally reserved for more severe cases (50 degrees or more). During surgery, the curve is corrected using a combination of fixation instruments and the patient's own bones. Often, a metal rod is placed on each vertebra of the spine to hold it in place for the rest of the patient's life.

It's important to note that each patient and each case of scoliosis is unique, so the appropriate treatment will depend on various factors. It is crucial to work with a spine specialist to determine the best treatment plan for each individual case, as each case is completely different from the other.

In general, the choice of treatment will depend on the severity of the spinal curvature, the patient's age, and other individual factors. If detected early, scoliosis can be successfully treated and further progression of the curve can be prevented.

THE CORSET

The choice of using a corset as a treatment for my scoliosis was a carefully considered decision made by my family and me after extensive research and discussions with various healthcare professionals, family members, and friends. There were several treatment options available to rectify the curvature of my spine, such as physical therapy and the use of corsets, but we chose the second one.

Initially, my family and I were concerned about the possibility of having surgery to correct my scoliosis. Surgery is a common treatment option for severe scoliosis, although it is not currently necessary in my case, and it requires a prolonged hospital stay and significant recovery time. Additionally, surgery carries inherent risks, such as infections, blood loss, and nerve injuries.

My orthopedic specialist suggested the use of a corset, which is an orthopedic device that is worn to restrict the movement of the spine and reduce the curvature. The corset is individually fitted to the shape of the spine and body and can be worn throughout the day and night, except during physical activity. (Initially, it was challenging to adapt to it, but eventually, I became more comfortable with it than without it, something that can sound crazy.)

My family and I extensively researched the option of using a brace and came across cases of other scoliosis patients who, along with their families, had chosen the same treatment. Through this research, we discovered that when used correctly and consistently, the corset can be a highly effective option for reducing or maintaining the curvature of the spine and preventing further progression in the future.

Furthermore, using a corset has numerous advantages over surgery. It does not carry the same level of risk of complications and does not require a prolonged hospital stay or significant recovery time. Therefore, it is worth trying the brace as a treatment option, as long as the curvature is not so severe that the medical team recommends otherwise initially.

Additionally, the brace can be adjusted and modified as my spine changes and as I grow, which means that the treatment can be adapted to my needs as I get older.

Finally, after considering all the options and consulting with medical professionals, my family and I decided that the corset was the best option for me. Although wearing it was not an easy solution, we realized that it was an effective way to treat my scoliosis and maintain hope that surgery would not be necessary.

In summary, the choice of using a corset as a treatment for my scoliosis has been a carefully considered decision made after extensive research and dialogue with doctors and other healthcare professionals. Although there are several treatment options available, we found that the corset, at that time and to this day, is the best option for me. It is effective and adaptable, and does not rule out the possibility of surgery if it becomes necessary in the future. It is important to note that surgery, being a much more invasive option with risks, is our last option.

THE REACTION OF MY FAMILY

Using a brace to treat scoliosis can have a significant impact on the life of a patient and their family. When I was diagnosed with scoliosis and the use of a brace was recommended, my family and I had many emotions and concerns in mind.

Firstly, there was concern about the effectiveness of the treatment. We wondered and still wonder if the brace would be sufficient to correct or maintain my spinal curvature, as we were also warned that reversing the curvature is very difficult. We know that the possibility of surgery is always present, although we hope that after all the sacrifice and discomfort that comes with wearing the brace, it will not be necessary.

Additionally, there was some anxiety related to the process of adapting to the corset . It was an unfamiliar device to us, and we did not know what it would be like to wear it. There were also concerns about how the corset would affect my daily comfort and quality of life. Would it be painful? Would it be restrictive? How would it impact my ability to engage in physical activities? How much discomfort could I tolerate? Would I be able to sleep with it on? There were many questions in my mind!

Another significant concern was the social aspect. As a teenager, I was worried about how the corset would look under my clothes, how others would see me, and how it would later modify my confidence in my appearance and self-esteem. We also wondered how my friends and classmates would react to knowing that I was using a corset (we all know how cruel people can be, especially certain teenagers). In this aspect, I have to say that everyone close to me was really understanding, so I would like to thank them from here.

Fortunately, I had and continue to have a lot of support from my family and friends during this tedious process. My parents were constantly checking how I felt with the corset and made sure it was properly adjusted and worn correctly, without causing skin abrasions or sores.

As I got used to the brace, I found that it was not as restrictive as I feared. Although it did feel uncomfortable at first, I learned to move more easily and found ways to adapt to the limitations of the brace. As my body became accustomed to the device, the pain and discomfort decreased, and I even reached a state of comfort while wearing the brace. It may seem unbelievable, but it becomes a part of you, and you even miss it when you have to go without it for hours due to some reason.

I also discovered that the corset did not significantly affect my ability to engage in physical activities, as there was no issue with removing the device for sports or occasional recreational activities.

As time went on, wearing the corset became a normal part of my daily life. It was no longer something that caused me concern, but simply another tool to maintain my health and prevent complications in the future, a fact that was also understood by everyone close to me.

Overall, although wearing it has its challenges, I am grateful for having made that decision. I hope it will help me avoid surgery and achieve better alignment of my spine. Furthermore, I learned to be more resilient and adapt to difficult situations. The support of my family and friends was also crucial in my process of adaptation and acceptance of the treatment.

4 - THE TREATMENT

In this chapter, we will focus on the process of treating my scoliosis using a corset and how my condition has evolved since I started this therapy. We will address topics such as the duration of the treatment, expectations of improvement, the results obtained, and the necessary medical follow-up to monitor the progression of my spinal curve. We will discover how the treatment has affected my daily life and what challenges I have faced during this process. Not only that, but we will also analyze how the support of my family and friends has been crucial in dealing with the ups and downs of the treatment. Through my story, I hope to provide valuable information to those facing a similar situation and help them understand what a scoliosis treatment implies.

DURATION OF TREATMENT

The duration of treatment for scoliosis with a corset varies depending on the degree of spinal curvature, the age of the patient, and other individual factors. In general, wearing it is expected for approximately 15 to 23 hours a day for several years, or until the patient has stopped growing, and the spinal curve has stopped progressing.

The duration of corset wearing may seem overwhelming at first, but it is important to remember that every hour spent wearing the brace is an hour working towards correcting the spinal curve. Additionally, the time wearing it can be divided throughout the day, making the treatment more manageable.

In some cases, adjustments to the duration of corset treatment can be made based on the progression of the spinal curve, which is what typically happens. If the curve stabilizes earlier than expected, the corset wearing time may be reduced. On the other hand, if the curve continues to progress, the wearing time may need to be increased or modifications to it may be necessary, as was the case for me.

The expectations of improvement also vary depending on each individual case. Generally, the primary goal of corset treatment is to prevent the spinal curve from getting worse and, in some cases, to correct it to some extent, although this is not guaranteed by using the device. Unfortunately, there are cases where no matter what is done to try to reduce the curve, it is not possible, as scoliosis is a physical condition that is still not well understood. The amount of correction that can be achieved depends on the initial degree of curvature and the age of the patient, among other factors.

In some cases, corset treatment may be the only one needed to manage scoliosis, especially if it is detected early and treatment begins at a young age. However, in other cases, the treatment may be only part of the treatment plan, and surgery may be considered if the spinal curve continues to progress or if the patient experiences severe symptoms.

It is important to note that while corset treatment can be effective in correcting or preventing the progression of scoliosis, it is not a cure. The patient may need to continue monitoring their spine throughout their lifetime to ensure that the curve does not progress again.

In summary, the duration of the treatment can vary, but generally, the patient is expected to wear it for approximately 15 to 23 hours a day for several years. Expectations of improvement also vary depending on the individual case, but the main goal is to prevent the curve from getting worse and, in some cases, to correct it to some extent. Corset treatment may be sufficient in some cases, but in others, it may be part of a broader treatment plan. It is crucial to remember that brace treatment is not a cure, and the patient may need to continue monitoring their spine throughout their lifetime.

5—THE CORSET

Welcome to Chapter 5 of my story, where I will share my experience using the two types of corsets mentioned earlier to correct my scoliosis.

As I grew older, my spinal curve got worse, which meant that my only treatment option was to use an orthopedic corset. This chapter will focus on the stage when the corset was introduced into my life and how my body and mind adapted to its daily use.

Firstly, I will explore how the corsets are fitted. Orthopedic corsets are custom-made, so it is crucial that the measurement and molding process is accurate to ensure their effectiveness. Next, I will explain how the corset works and how it helps correct the curve in my spine. Although wearing the corset was an uncomfortable and restrictive experience, I discovered that over time, it helped me maintain better posture and preserve the curvature of my back.

Lastly, I will talk about how I felt when using the corset for the first time and how I adapted to its daily use. Although it was challenging at first, I found ways to make it more comfortable and manageable in my everyday life. I will also share some of my concerns and fears about using a corset, as well as the benefits and challenges I experienced along the way.

HOW THE CORSET IS ADJUSTED

The process of creating and fitting the corset was a significant step in my scoliosis treatment. It involved measurement and molding to ensure that the corset fit perfectly to my body. In this chapter, I will describe in detail what the corset fitting process was like for me and how the corset adapted to my body to provide effective correction of the curve in my spine. It's worth mentioning that I went through this process twice because my therapist believed that changing the type of corset used would be effective.

THE FIRST CORSET

The first step of the corset fitting process was taking measurements. My scoliosis specialist therapist measured my body from the waist to the upper and lower parts of my torso. Measurements were also taken around my rib cage and hips to gain a precise understanding of my body shape and size. These measurements were used to create a customized mold that would fit me perfectly.

Once the measurements were taken, a plaster cast of my trunk was made. The cast was created by having me stand for nearly an hour while orthopedic professionals wrapped strips of plaster around my body to mold the corset. The idea behind this was to have the plaster mold replicate my body exactly so that the corset would fit me perfectly.

After the mold was made, it was sent to a company specializing in custom corset manufacturing. The mold of my body was used to create the corset in a lab. The corset was made from thermoplastic material, which means it was heated in hot water and molded into a specific shape.

Once the corset was fabricated, I had to attend several appointments to have it properly adjusted. During the fitting appointments, the orthopedist and medical staff helped me put on the corset and adjusted it according to the necessary specifications to provide the most positive effect on my spine and posture. The corset was precisely fitted to ensure it was tight enough to correct or at least prevent the progression of my spinal curvature, yet comfortable enough for me to wear for extended periods of time.

The corset fitting process was a novel and interesting experience for me. It was a bit uncomfortable to stand with the plaster wrapped around my body for the molding process, but the medical staff was very kind and understanding. It was also exciting to see the mold of my body and how it was used to create a personalized corset.

Once the corset was properly fitted, I noticed a significant difference in my posture and how my body felt overall. The corset provided solid support to my back and allowed me to stand and walk with a more upright posture. I was also pleasantly surprised to find that the corset wasn't as uncomfortable to wear as I had expected. I thought it would be highly restrictive and limit my movement, but it wasn't the case.

Overall, the corset fitting process was a success for me. Although it may seem a bit intimidating at first, the medical staff and the technology behind the corset assured me that I was in good hands. The measurements and personalized manufacturing pleasantly surprised me and gave fascinating results. I would also like to emphasize that the process of starting to wear the corset can be quite challenging, especially in the beginning.

HOW THE CORSET WORKS

The corset is a supportive device that is worn around the torso to help correct the curvature of the spine. It works by applying pressure to the curved areas of the spine, helping to straighten them and maintain a more upright position. The corset can be used to treat scoliosis in children and teenagers, and is most commonly used in children who are still growing and developing.

The corset is carefully adjusted to fit the patient's body and is molded as the spine evolves or the patient grows (in my case). The molding process is done using thermoplastic materials, which are heated and molded to the shape of the patient's body. Once molded, the corset is secured in place and worn every day for several hours. The number of hours depends entirely on the patient and can range from 12 hours in milder cases to 24 hours in more significant cases. Personally, I had to wear the corset for 23 hours a day because my curve was quite significant.

As I mentioned, the way the corset works to correct the curvature of the spine is by applying pressure to the curved areas. By applying pressure, a straightening effect is achieved, helping to align the spine. Additionally, the corset also helps maintain the spine in a straighter position, which helps prevent further curvature. In cases of an S-shaped curve, two pressure zones are usually used, whereas in cases of a C-shaped curve (most cases), a single pressure zone is typically used, although I must reiterate that this varies in each case.

The corset can also help alleviate the pain and discomfort associated with scoliosis, as was the case for me. By applying pressure to the curved areas of the spine, tension in the muscles and ligaments of the back is reduced, which can relieve pain and discomfort. Furthermore, the corset also helps improve posture and spinal alignment, which can help prevent additional health problems in the future.

The use of the corset is an effective way to treat scoliosis in children and adolescents. However, it is important to note that the corset is NOT A CURE for scoliosis. Instead, it is used to help correct the curvature of the spine and prevent further deviation. Additionally, the use of the corset may require significant commitment, as it needs to be worn every day for several hours, and sometimes the curve continues desenvoluping, making the corset less effective.

Overall, the corset is an effective and safe treatment option for scoliosis. It helps correct the curvature of the spine and prevent further deviation, while alleviating the pain and discomfort associated with the condition. While the process of fitting and molding the corset may be somewhat uncomfortable at first, many people quickly adapt to wearing the corset daily and find that it significantly improves their quality of life.

So, from here, I encourage all of you who are currently unsure about whether to use a corset, whether due to discomfort, fear, or simply the opinions of others, to first think about your health.

HOW WEARING A CORSET FEELS

Wearing a corset has been a significant part of my life, and in this chapter, I would like to share my experience of what it's like to wear it, how I adapted to it, and the different emotions I went through over time.

When I received my first corset, I remember feeling overwhelmed and scared. I wasn't sure how I would cope with wearing such a large and heavy device all the time. The process of putting it on was also a bit uncomfortable at first, as I had to stand for a long time while it was measured and molded to fit my body. But as time went on, I realized it wasn't as bad as I had initially thought.

The corset I was given was quite rigid and made of hard plastic, but it was designed to be as comfortable as possible. It was adjusted with straps around the rib cage and waist, allowing for some flexibility and movement in the trunk while still keeping my spine straight and in the correct position. Initially, I felt a bit self-conscious and clumsy as I got used to wearing it, but I quickly realized that it helped me maintain a straighter posture and improved my breathing and lung capacity, which motivated me to continue using the device.

Another concern of mine was how the corset would look under my clothes. However, I soon discovered that with the right clothing, it could be hidden quite well. I chose to wear a tight-fitting cotton shirt underneath the device to prevent rubbing, as well as loose-fitting sweatshirts and high-waisted pants to minimize the visibility of the corset. Surprisingly, most people didn't even notice that I was wearing it, although if I wore slightly tight shirts or short-sleeved shirts, some people would notice it.

As time went on, I started to feel more comfortable with the corset and appreciate its benefits. It helped me maintain my posture, which in turn relieved pressure on my spine and reduced the back pain I often experienced. I also felt more confident and comfortable with myself, disregarding the stares or opinions of others, as I knew I was doing the right thing to correct my scoliosis.

Despite all that, there were still moments when I felt frustrated and limited by the corset. However, despite these limitations, I decided to continue wearing the corset because it was working. The results of my X-rays initially showed that the curve of my spine hadn't worsened, which was quite a positive outcome.

I had been using the device for about two years, and I believed that the device was doing an excellent job of correcting my spine. But a harsh reality hit me when my physical therapist informed me that my curve had worsened from around 35 degrees to about 45 degrees in less than a year. I was shocked to hear this news because I had been putting in all my effort to wear the brace and follow all the instructions I had been given. I wondered how it was possible for the curve to have become even worse, and I felt frustrated and discouraged.

Not only that, but I was explained that my curvature had shifted to the thoracic region, making it more dangerous and difficult to treat. According to my orthopedic specialist, the lower part of the curve hadn't worsened, but due to growth, the deviation had shifted to the upper part of my back.

SECOND CORSET

My physiotherapist and I debated whether I should continue using the corset or not because it hadn't been effective. They explained that sometimes corsets don't function as they should, or patients don't use them properly, and there are many factors that can influence the progress of scoliosis. We decided that it would be best to switch to a new device and try to stabilize the curve and prevent further deterioration.

My orthopedist decided that the best type of corset would be a "Milwaukee" one, which was much more uncomfortable to wear because it had a chin support and a back support attached to the head. This was a setback because unlike the previous corset I had, the Milwaukee one was much more restrictive, covering more parts of the body, and had more adjustments and straps.

The moment you receive the news can be frustrating, as you may believe that the progress is not going well, that you're regressing, and getting closer to the surgery you desperately want to avoid. However, you resign yourself and move forward, finding the necessary strength because you understand that there is no other alternative, and you continue to have faith that everything will turn out well.

I had to readjust to a new corset and start over; the first few days were tough. I remember not even being able to get into the car because I could hardly bend with it on. My parents were also shocked when they saw it, when we went to pick it up from the orthopedic center, and they conducted the initial tests and adjustments. They told me to gradually adapt to it, to start wearing it for short periods of time, to try stretching in bed, and so on.

The process of making a new corset was long and complicated, but it was worth it. They took many measurements, and a 3D scan of my trunk was done to ensure the corset fit perfectly on my body. The new device was much more comfortable than the previous one and didn't interfere as much with my daily life since I didn't have to wear it to school. I learned how to use it properly and made sure to follow all the instructions from my physiotherapist.

One small piece of advice I would like to give to people who are about to start using a corset is not to fear the device or the opinions of others about their physical condition, and, above all, to ask any questions they may have to both professionals and their family.

THE EXPECTATIONS FOR IMPROVENT

The expectations for improvement are a significant aspect for anyone dealing with scoliosis and seeking treatment to improve their condition. In my case, when I was diagnosed with scoliosis, one of the recommended treatments was the use of a corset. During the treatment process, I had very low expectations about how the device could improve my posture and alleviate my pain.

As time went on, my expectations about the corset started to change. Initially, I only hoped that it would help me experience less pain, but I soon realized that it could do much more than that. I began to see the corset as a tool to improve my posture and my overall quality of life.

However, there were also challenges associated with wearing the device. The corset is uncomfortable to wear for long periods, especially in hot weather. I also found it difficult to find clothing that fit well with the corset and was comfortable to wear, as I explained in more detail in the previous chapter.

Despite these challenges, I continue to wear the device and work hard to achieve the results I hope for. I make sure to follow my doctor's instructions and properly care for the corset to maximize its effectiveness.

Although there have been times when I felt a bit discouraged, I also realize that this is an opportunity to learn more about my body and my condition. I have asked many questions to my physiotherapist and conducted research on scoliosis and treatment options. I discovered that there are many different types of corsets, and some are more effective than others for certain types of curves, which led us to decide that it was best to create a custom-made device for me, tailored to my body and specific curve.

In addition to using the new corset, I also started implementing other changes in my life to help improve my condition. I began going to the gym, strengthening the muscles in my back, and improving my posture in my daily activities.

I learned that scoliosis is a condition that requires a unique approach to treatment for each patient. There is no one-size-fits-all solution, and each person needs to work with their medical team to find the best treatment options for their specific situation. I discovered that scoliosis not only affects the spine but the entire body, and it is important to address all areas to achieve overall improvement.

I also learned the importance of having a positive mindset and not allowing scoliosis to define me. Initially, I felt frustrated and limited by my condition, but after working with my medical team and making lifestyle changes, I began to feel more in control and optimistic about my future. I learned that scoliosis didn't have to restrict my activities or goals, and that I could continue doing the things I loved with a bit more care and attention.

In summary, the chapter of my story about changing corsets was a pivotal moment in my battle against scoliosis. I learned that scoliosis is a complex condition that requires a unique approach to treatment, and working with a trusted medical team is essential. I also learned the importance of making lifestyle changes and having a positive mindset to achieve overall improvement in my health and well-being.

6 - THE HIGHTS AND LOWS

In this chapter, we will explore the ups and downs I face in my daily life while dealing with scoliosis and the corset. While the treatment can be effective in correcting the curvature of my spine, it also presents challenges that impact my everyday life. In this chapter, I will discuss how the corset has changed my routine and the challenges I sometimes encounter, as well as the strategies I have developed to cope with them. I will also explore how my mood can fluctuate based on how I feel about scoliosis and the device. By sharing my personal experiences, I hope to offer a deeper insight into the emotional and practical ups and downs that can arise during scoliosis treatment.

DAILY CHALLENGES

One of the biggest daily challenges I have faced since starting to wear the corset is difficulty sleeping. Initially, it was uncomfortable and difficult to sleep with it on. The corset feels tight and restrictive, and I couldn't find a comfortable sleeping position. Additionally, the device makes it harder to take deep breaths. But fortunately, as I mentioned in previous chapters, I gradually got used to wearing it, and eventually, it became much easier to sleep with the device than without it.

Another significant challenge is limited mobility. The corset restricts my ability to move freely, which can be uncomfortable and restrictive in daily life. Even simple tasks like sitting, bending, or lifting objects can be challenging or uncomfortable with the device on. Additionally, it can affect my posture, which sometimes makes me feel clumsy and off-balance when walking.

Furthermore, clothing can be an issue when wearing the corset. Initially, it was challenging to find clothes that fit comfortably over the device without being too tight or restrictive. I had to change my style of dressing and look for looser and more comfortable garments to wear with it.

Another challenge I faced was concern about appearance. Initially, I felt very self-conscious about how the corset made my body look, and I worried that others would notice the bulges the device created throughout my torso. I had to work on overcoming this concern and learn to feel more comfortable with my body and appearance, and luckily, I succeeded.

To confront these challenges, I developed some strategies that helped me cope with the daily use of the corset. One thing I did was establish a daily routine for putting on and taking off the device. I learned to do it efficiently and find ways to make the process faster and less uncomfortable by creating habits.

I also made adjustments in my lifestyle and daily activities to accommodate the corset. For example, I learned to sit and move differently to avoid discomfort and restriction. I also started exercising more, primarily aiming to help prevent pain and injuries related to its usage.

Finally, I learned to accept and love my body despite the device and its limitations. I learned to dress in a way that made me feel comfortable and confident, and worked to change my perspective on my appearance and body. Although wearing a corset can be challenging, I discovered that with time and practice, it becomes a more manageable part of daily life. Wearing the device also made me understand why its usage was crucial in my condition and the great work it was doing.

HOW I FIGHT AGAINST THE CORSET

In this subchapter, I will describe my own strategies for dealing with the corset, as well as the emotions that sometimes arise during the treatment.

When I started wearing the device, it took me some time to get used to the feeling of having something so tight around my trunk. At first, I felt like it was a heavy burden that prevented me from doing simple things like bending down to tie my shoes or sitting comfortably in a chair. But over time, I learned to make adjustments and find alternative ways of doing things.

One of the first things I did was research the best way to dress with the corset. I discovered that loose and comfortable clothing is the best option to minimize discomfort. I also avoid wearing non-cotton shirts or anything that could rub against the skin under the brace and cause irritation. Not only that, but I learned to be strategic in choosing my daily activities as well. For example, I avoid going to crowd places or standing for long periods, as these can increase discomfort.

Another thing I did to improve my experience with the device was to try out various methods and techniques for activities that became difficult or uncomfortable with the corset, such as tying shoelaces or sitting for extended periods. Through this experimentation, I managed to find ways to perform these activities without any discomfort or pain. It took considerable time and effort to discover these methods, but I can say that it was definitely worth it.

Acceptance has been one of the main strategies I have used. Accepting that I have scoliosis and need to wear a corset has been crucial in dealing with its use. Initially, I was resistant to accepting that I had a condition that required wearing it. However, over time, I learned that accepting my condition was the only way to move forward and find ways to cope with the device.

Communication has also been an effective strategy for me. Talking to friends and family about my condition and the use of the corset has helped me feel more comfortable and less isolated. Additionally, I have reached out to other corset-wearing patients through social media and forums to seek support and advice on how to deal with the device.

Distraction has also proven to be a helpful strategy. Instead of focusing on the discomfort and physical limitations I experience with it, I try to engage in other activities to distract myself. I focus on hobbies, read books, listen to music, or watch movies to keep my mind occupied and distracted from the device.

One solution I found for dealing with the corset was wearing seamless cotton shirts. Initially, I was unsure of what type of clothing would be the best option to wear with the device, but after experimenting with different fabrics and styles, I discovered that soft, seamless cotton shirts were the most comfortable. Seams and rough fabrics can irritate the skin and cause additional discomfort. The soft and breathable fabric of cotton shirts also helped keep my skin cool and dry, reducing sweating and eliminating chafing.

Lastly, it's important to remember that it's okay to feel sad, frustrated, or upset about having to wear a brace. Recognizing and accepting these emotions is a crucial step in being able to cope with them. Talking to friends, family, or people who are going through a similar situation can help process these emotions and find healthy ways to manage them.

In summary, there are many strategies that can be used to cope with wearing a corset and the emotions that arise. Acceptance, communication, distraction, therapy, planning, and organization are just some of the strategies that can be helpful. Each person can find their own way of dealing with wearing a brace, and it's indispensable to remember that it's okay to feel sad or frustrated from time to time.

THE GOODS AND THE BAD DAYS

Dealing with a chronic medical condition like scoliosis and wearing a corset can indeed be exhausting, both physically and emotionally. It's important to acknowledge and validate the challenges you face in your daily life and treatment journey.

On good days, when you feel confident and secure with your device on, it's a positive experience. You can walk with a straight posture, take pride in your appearance, and appreciate the corset as a tool that helps correct the curvature of your spine and improve your long-term health. These days empower you to face challenges with a positive and optimistic attitude.

However, there are also bad days when you may feel trapped in your device. It can be difficult to find clothing that fits comfortably over it, which can lead to discomfort and a lack of confidence. You might feel self-conscious about your appearance and find it challenging to socialize with others without feeling entirely at ease.

Additionally, the prolonged use of the corset can be painful and exhausting. There are days when you experience back pain and feel uncomfortable and limited in your movements.

As you spend more time wearing the device, you learn to recognize and cope with these emotional ups and downs. One effective strategy is to surround yourself with understanding and supportive individuals who comprehend your situation and provide emotional support. Your family and friends have been a great source of support throughout your treatment journey, offering encouragement and motivation that helps you maintain a positive outlook even on the toughest days.

Engaging in physical activities, such as going to the gym, has also been a helpful strategy in coping with wearing the corset. These activities help relieve stress and muscular tension, contributing to improved mood and emotional well-being. It's important to discuss with your therapist and agree upon, removing it when necessary to engage in physical activity comfortably.

Overall, the emotional ups and downs you experience during your scoliosis treatment with a corset are a significant part of your journey. While the device is an effective treatment for correcting the curve of your spine, it also has a profound impact on your daily life and emotional well-being. Remember to prioritize self-care and seek support from loved ones as you navigate these challenges.

7 - THE SOCIAL LIFE

In this chapter, we will explore how scoliosis and the corset have affected my social life. From the moment I received the diagnosis, I knew that my life would never be the same. My relationships with friends and classmates would change, and I would have to adapt to a different lifestyle. In this chapter, I will share my experiences and challenges, as well as the strategies I have used to continue enjoying social life despite the limitations imposed by scoliosis and the device. I will also discuss others' opinions, how they react when they see it, and how I feel about it. I hope that by sharing my story, I can help others who are going through a similar time and perhaps even provide some inspiration and hope.

CHANGES IN MY SOCIAL LIFE

First and foremost, the corset became something that was always present in my life and influenced all my social activities. For example, I would sometimes feel self-conscious when going out with friends because I knew I would have to explain why I was wearing the device and how it affected my mobility. Even the simplest activities, like sitting in a chair or lying on the sofa, became more complicated due to the restricted movement of the corset. This also affected my ability to participate in sports and other physical activities, making me feel isolated and different from my friends who could do these things with ease.

Furthermore, I realized that some people simply did not understand my situation. I often received well-intentioned but insensitive comments about my appearance or about how it must be uncomfortable to wear a corset all day. Even my close friends sometimes seemed to forget that I had to wear the device and were surprised when I had to make adjustments in our activities to accommodate my limitations.

Another change I noticed was that I sometimes felt excluded from conversations or activities because of having to wear it. I felt like I had to somehow give up on doing certain things to maintain my treatment and medical care, and that was sometimes difficult to accept.

However, there were also moments when my friends and classmates showed their support and understanding. Some offered to help me make adjustments in our activities to ensure I felt comfortable, and others simply listened to my concerns and offered words of encouragement. I also discovered that there were online groups and communities on social media dedicated to people with scoliosis and other medical conditions, and I could connect with people who were going through similar situations.

Overall, the changes in my social life due to scoliosis and the corset have been a challenge, but also an opportunity to learn and grow. It has led me to be more compassionate and understanding towards others who may be going through medical or emotional difficulties, and it has also taught me to be more aware of my own needs and limitations. While there have been ups and downs in my social life due to scoliosis and the device, I am grateful for the opportunity to face these challenges and grow as a person.

THE OPINION OF THE OTHERS

The opinions of others can have a significant impact on how we feel about ourselves and our circumstances. For someone wearing a corset due to scoliosis, the reactions of those around them can be a sensitive issue. Others may struggle to understand the need for the device or hold biases regarding its appearance. In this section, we will explore how people react when they see it and how it can affect someone who wears it.

It is natural to feel a bit nervous when showing the corset to others for the first time. Many people fear being judged or having uncomfortable questions asked. Children and teenagers wearing, they may be especially vulnerable to feeling embarrassed or different from their peers or close ones. It is important to remember that the device is a necessary medical device and there is nothing to be ashamed of. Over time, many patients (like myself) find that they become more comfortable discussing their brace and condition with others. This is because they accept the condition and no longer see it as a major issue.

People's reactions often depend on their prior knowledge of scoliosis and corsets. Those who have some prior knowledge or who have friends or family members who have worn one may have a better understanding of why it is used and be more compassionate. However, for those unfamiliar with the condition, the device may appear strange or unfamiliar. Some people may ask curious questions or make inappropriate comments without realizing the impact they can have on the patient.

In some cases, others may have a negative reaction towards the corset and its appearance. Some people may feel uncomfortable or disgusted upon seeing the device. This can lead to cruel comments or even teasing. I must say that fortunately, I did not receive any teasing or negative comments about it, so I consider myself really lucky. For those who are subjected to these behaviors, it can be challenging to maintain a positive and understanding attitude. In these cases, it is important to remember that the corset is a necessary medical device and has nothing to do with personal appearance.

Essentially, the way others react to the device can vary widely. Some may be understanding and compassionate, while others may be cruel or ignorant. For those wearing corsets, it is crucial to remember that their health and well-being are the number one priority, and they should not feel ashamed or uncomfortable about it. It is also relevant for friends, family, and others surrounding the patient to make an effort to be understanding and compassionate, and to ask questions in a respectful and considerate manner. The conclusion I would like to reach is that, together, we can work to increase awareness about scoliosis and corsets and also help patients feel more comfortable and supported in their treatment process.

THE SOCIAL ACTIVITIES

Scoliosis and wearing a corset can make certain social activities challenging, but that doesn't mean you have to give up on your favorite hobbies and social events. With some planning and adaptations, you can continue to do fun things and hang out with your friends.

Here are some strategies I have found helpful in continuing to enjoy social life while wearing my device to treat my scoliosis.

Choose comfortable activities:
When planning a social activity, it's important to choose something that is comfortable to do with the corset. For example, if I'm planning a hiking outing, I make sure the trail is flat and not inclined, as this can make walking with it is more difficult.

Communicate my needs to my friends:
Friends may not know how to help us navigate the corset and scoliosis, so it's crucial to communicate my needs to them. If I need to rest or sit during an activity, I let them know.

Plan ahead:
Planning ahead can make social activities much easier to manage. I always try to plan everything in advance to see if I can do it with the device or not and how it will affect what I'm going to do.

Wear comfortable clothing:
Wearing comfortable clothing is key to feeling at ease while wearing it. I look for loose and comfortable clothing that doesn't fit too tightly. Seamless cotton shirts are a good choice as they don't rub against the skin and allow for airflow.

Find enjoyable activities to do at home:
There are days when I simply don't feel up to going out, so I find fun activities to do at home. I can play video games, read, write, watch movies, or play board games.

Take advantage of exercise opportunities:
Exercise can be challenging when wearing a corset, so I take off the device for a brief period of time to engage in the activity I want. For example, I always remove the device when going to the gym. This may sound unreasonable, but it's actually beneficial, as it helps strengthen the back and improve posture.

In summary, although the corset and scoliosis may present some challenges in social life, they don't have to prevent me from doing fun things with my friends and family. By planning ahead, communicating my needs, and finding comfortable activities, I can continue to enjoy my social life while managing the scoliosis.

8 - THE ADJUSTMENTS OF THE DEVICE

The process of treating scoliosis with a corset can be long and challenging. Once treatment has begun, it's important to understand that the device is not a permanent solution and will require periodic adjustments to ensure it continues to be effective in correcting the spinal curve.

In this chapter, we will discuss the process of it adjustments, including the frequency of adjustments and how the process is carried out. We will also address a crucial topic, which could be considered the dark side of adjustments: pain. It is common to experience pain after corset adjustments, but there are strategies to help manage it.

The device adjustment is an essential part of the treatment, and it is crucial for patients to be informed about what to expect during this process. Throughout this chapter, I will try to share valuable information to help patients feel more prepared and comfortable during adjustments.

FREQUENCY OF ADJUSTMENTS

Adjustments are necessary to ensure the corset fits properly as the body grows and develops. The frequency of adjustments varies depending on the patient, the severity of the curve, and the type of it used. In my case, the device was only adjusted when I noticed that I had grown and felt the chin support was somewhat low.

Doctors and orthotists usually recommend corset adjustments every 3 to 6 months. However, this can vary depending on age and the degree of curvature. Younger patients and those with more severe curves may require more frequent adjustments. During periods of rapid growth, adjustments may be necessary more often as the body changes quickly, as was the case for me.

In my experience, corset adjustments were a regular part of my treatment. At first, I was nervous about the adjustments because I didn't know what to expect. However, after a few adjustments, I got used to the process and started feeling more comfortable during the medical appointments.

It's important for patients to regularly schedule appointments with their doctors for adjustments. Scoliosis treatment is a long-term process, and thorough supervision is necessary to ensure the treatment is working properly. If necessary adjustments are skipped, the device can lose its effectiveness, and the spinal curve may worsen, rendering all the effort in vain.

In summary, the frequency of adjustments varies depending on the patient and the severity of the curve. Patients should regularly schedule appointments with their doctors and orthotists to ensure the corset fits properly, and that scoliosis treatment is working effectively.

HOW THE CORSET IS ADJUSTED

The process of corset adjustment can vary from person to person, depending on the type of it and the severity of scoliosis. In my case, my current corset is a full-body Milwaukee, which means it covers from my neck to my hips and has straps to adjust the compression in different parts of my trunk.

Before each adjustment, I have to remove the device and wear a seamless undershirt to protect my skin. Then, my orthopedist measures my spine and the curvature of my scoliosis to determine if any changes need to be made to it.

Adjusting the corset involves tightening or loosening the straps in different areas of the device to help correct the curvature of my spine and prevent it from worsening. It also involves raising the chin support to ensure proper neck alignment. Sometimes, this means using pads or adding/removing certain elements to accommodate my growth.

The adjustment process itself is not painful, but it can be uncomfortable and requires some skill to properly position the straps. During the adjustment, I often feel a bit constrained, which is normal given the compression of the device. It's uncomfortable, but I hope it will be worth it.

However, the adjustment process is only one part of the journey. After each adjustment, my body needs time to adapt to the changes and get used to the corset. I may feel a bit more uncomfortable or stiff during the first few days after the adjustment, but after a few days of wearing it, my body gets accustomed to it again.

It's important to mention that the corset adjustment process is crucial for the success of scoliosis treatment. Regular adjustment appointments and modifications as my body grows are essential. This ensures that the treatment is working effectively to correct my spine and prevent the curve from worsening over time.

Overall, while the process of adjustment is not always comfortable, I know it is necessary for my health and to prevent my scoliosis from worsening. I've learned to be patient and trust the process, knowing that each adjustment is a step closer to correcting my spine and improving my quality of life in the future.

THE PAIN ASSOCIATED WITH THE CORSET

One of the most challenging aspects of wearing a corset to treat scoliosis is the pain associated with regular adjustments. Every time I need an adjustment in my device, I know that I'm about to go through a painful process. Although the pain is temporary and alleviates after a few days, the adjustment is a difficult part of the treatment that cannot be ignored.

The process of adjustment sometimes involves visiting the orthopedist and spending a significant amount of time in the clinic. First, the doctor examines me to assess the curve of my spine and determine how much the device needs to be adjusted. Then, the corset is removed to allow the orthopedist to make the necessary modifications. Sometimes, the corset needs to stay at the orthotics facility for a few days, and when the orthopedist is done adjusting the device, my family is notified to come and pick up it.

Even though it may seem strange, the days I don't sleep with the device because it's being adjusted, I feel like a part of me is missing, and I feel really uncomfortable. This is because my body has become habituated to having the shape of the corset. I know that the adjustment is necessary to keep my spinal curve under control, but I can't help feeling a great sense of emptiness inside me every time I go through this process.

After the orthopedist finishes making the adjustments, the device is placed back on my body. Often, I feel significant discomfort and pain as my body adapts to the new shape of the corset. There are times when the discomfort is so intense that I can't concentrate on other things while wearing it. It is also common to experience back and neck pain after an adjustment, as my body tries to adapt to the new position of my spine.

Despite all the pain and discomfort I experience after the adjustments, I know that it's important to take care of myself and do everything possible to minimize the pain and discomfort. Some of the strategies I use to manage the pain after adjustments include:

Rest and relaxation:
After an adjustment, I try to take a few days to rest and relax as much as possible. This helps reduce the pain and discomfort in my body and allows me to recover more quickly.

Exercise:
I also engage in exercise to help my body adapt to the new shape of the brace and to try to distract myself. Going to the gym is particularly helpful for me to strengthen my body and reduce pain.

Open communication with my orthopedist:

If I experience persistent or unbearable pain after an adjustment, I make sure to communicate it to my orthopedist. They may be able to provide additional guidance or make further adjustments to alleviate the discomfort.

Pain management techniques:
I also utilize pain management techniques such as applying heat or cold packs, taking nonprescription pain medications as recommended by my healthcare provider, or using relaxation techniques to help alleviate the pain and discomfort.

It's important to remember that each individual's experience with corset adjustments and associated pain may vary. It's crucial to consult with a healthcare professional for personalized advice and guidance throughout the treatment process.

9 - THE OVERCOMING

In this chapter, we will explore how it is possible to overcome the challenges presented by scoliosis and the corset, and how one can learn to live positively with this condition.

Firstly, we will discuss learning and how I have come to understand and accept scoliosis and the device in my daily life. There may be times when the process seems overwhelming and difficult, but with time and patience, it can be possible to learn to live effectively with scoliosis.

Next, we will examine long-term goals and how scoliosis and the corset can impact them. Goals can vary from personal goals to professional goals, and scoliosis and the device may present obstacles on the path to their achievement. However, it is possible to find solutions to overcome these challenges and achieve our goals.

Lastly, we will talk about acceptance and how I have come to accept my condition and how I feel about it. Acceptance can be a difficult process and take time, but it is important to remember that scoliosis and wearing a corset do not define anyone. Learning to accept our condition and being positive about it can lead to a more fulfilling and happy life.

In summary, this chapter will explore how it is possible to overcome the challenges associated with scoliosis and the device, and how one can learn to live effectively with this condition. We will discuss learning, long-term goals, and acceptance, and we hope that this information provides a positive perspective on how we can effectively live our lives with this condition.

THE LEARNING

Living with scoliosis and wearing a corset can seem overwhelming at first. When I received my scoliosis diagnosis and started wearing it, I had no idea how I was going to cope with it. However, over time, I learned to live with the device and scoliosis, and today I can say that I have become an expert.

Learning to live with the corset and scoliosis involves several aspects. First and foremost, I learned about the anatomy of the spine and how it is affected by scoliosis. I learned about the curvature of the spine, the rotation of the vertebrae, and how this can impact my body. I also learned how the device works to correct my curvature and prevent it from worsening.

Furthermore, I learned how to properly wear it. Initially, putting on and adjusting the corset was quite a challenge that required significant assistance. But over time, I learned how to do it effectively. I learned how to position the pads correctly to avoid pressure points on my body, and how to adjust the straps to achieve the appropriate level of compression and spinal realignment.

Another important aspect was learning how to care for the device and keep it clean and in good condition. I learned to inspect the pads and straps for signs of wear and to replace them as needed.

I also learned how to incorporate the corset into my daily life. Not only that, but I learned to dress appropriately to avoid chafing and pressure points on my body. I learned how to sit properly with the device and avoid certain movements that could affect its position. Additionally, a crucial aspect was learning to sleep with it and find a comfortable position that allowed me to rest well.

In summary, learning to live with the corset and scoliosis involved learning about the anatomy of my body, how to wear and care for it, and how to incorporate it into my daily life. It was a continuous learning process that took time and dedication, but fortunately, it allowed me to live comfortably.

Learning also involved learning to deal with the emotions that arise from wearing a corset and living with scoliosis. I often felt frustrated and down, especially when facing pains or discomfort related to the device. But I learned to maintain a positive attitude and focus on the positive aspects of my life. I also learned to seek support from my family, friends, and online communities.

In conclusion, learning to live with the device and scoliosis was not easy, but it was an invaluable learning experience. It allowed me to develop practical skills to take care of my body and my health, and it also taught me to fight against my negative emotions. Although living with a chronic medical condition can be challenging, I am grateful for everything I have learned and how I have grown through this experience.

THE ACCEPTATION

Learning to accept a chronic health condition can be a difficult and challenging process. When I was diagnosed with scoliosis and told that I needed to wear acorset, I initially felt scared. I wondered how I was going to deal with this for the next years of my life, and if I would ever be able to accept my condition.

However, over time, I learned to accept my scoliosis condition and wearing it. I learned that acceptance is not a bad thing, but rather a positive attitude towards my situation. Here are some things I learned about accepting my condition and how I feel about it:

Seeking support:
One of the most important things I learned is that I was not alone. I sought out online support groups to connect with other people going through the same thing as me. This helped me realize that I was not the only one and that there were others who were in the same situation.

Embracing the ups and downs:
Accepting my condition meant accepting that there would be good days and bad days. There would be days when I would feel comfortable with the corsets and others when I would feel uncomfortable or limited. I learned not to accuse myself for feeling this way and to take time to take care of myself when needed.

Finding ways to express myself:
Acceptance also meant finding ways to express my personality and who I am despite . I started looking for shirts that I could wear with the device and other things that could help me feel more comfortable and confident. I discovered that even with it, I could still be myself.

Focusing on what I can do:
I also learned to focus on what I could change rather than what I couldn't. I learned to find activities that I could do with the corset, and discovered that I could still do many of the things I enjoyed before my diagnosis.

Gratitude for what I have:
Finally, I learned to be grateful for what I have instead of lamenting what I don't have. I learned to be thankful for my health and for the support of my family and friends. I learned that acceptance doesn't mean I have to be happy all the time, but that I can find happiness even in difficult circumstances.

In summary, learning to accept my scoliosis condition and wearing the corset was a challenging but worthwhile process. I learned to seek support, embrace the ups and downs, find ways to express myself, focus on what I can change, and be grateful for what I have. I learned that acceptance is not a bad thing but a positive attitude towards my situation. Today, I can confidently say that I have come to accept my condition, and I am grateful for the strength and personal growth I have gained through this process.

10 - THE REFLEXION

Welcome to Chapter 10 of this book, titled "Reflection." In this chapter, I will reflect on my experience with scoliosis and the corset, share tips for those going through a similar situation, and explain why I decided to write this book and share my story with others.

Reflexion is an important process where one looks back and ponders on their life. In my case, looking back on my experience with scoliosis and the device has allowed me to see how far I have come and how I have learned and grown through this experience. From diagnosis to acceptance, it has been a journey filled with emotional ups and downs, adjustments, and long-term goals. But, upon reflexion, I can see how I have found ways to adapt and overcome the challenges that have come my way.

In addition to personal reflection, I also want to share some tips I have learned throughout my experience. I understand that every experience is different, but I hope that by sharing my advice, I can help in some way or another those who may be going through a similar situation. These tips include how to cope with the pain and discomfort of the corset, how to talk to friends and family about the condition, and how to maintain a positive attitude during challenges.

Finally, I will discuss why I decided to write this book and share my story with others. By writing this book and sharing my experience, I hope to be able to help others who may feel the same and let them know that they are not alone.

In summary, in this chapter, I will reflect on my experience with scoliosis and the corset, share tips for those going through a similar situation, and explain why I decided to write this book and share my story with others. I hope that this chapter can be helpful and encouraging to those going through a similar situation.

LOOKING BACK

Scoliosis and wearing a brace have been challenging in my life, but they have also provided opportunities for growth and learning. Through this experience, I have learned to value my health and well-being, accept my condition, and seek the emotional support I need. I have also developed qualities such as compassion and empathy towards others facing difficulties.

If I could give advice to those going through a similar situation, I would encourage them to seek emotional support from the beginning. Openly talking to friends, family, or seeking support groups can help alleviate the feeling of isolation and provide the necessary support to face the challenges. Additionally, try to accept your condition and do not be ashamed of it. Remember that your condition does not define you as a person, and there are many other valuable and meaningful things in life.

Focusing on small victories and learning to appreciate the things that can still be done is another important key. Despite the limitations, it is possible to find activities that bring joy and satisfaction. Furthermore, practicing self-compassion and maintaining a positive attitude can make a significant difference in how you face the situation.

In conclusion, scoliosis and wearing a brace have left a profound impact on my life. Through this experience, I have learned to value my health, accept my condition, and seek the necessary support. I have also developed qualities such as compassion and empathy towards others. If you are going through a similar situation, remember that you are not alone, and there are resources and support available. Maintain a positive attitude and find ways to enjoy the things you can still do. Your story and experience can inspire and help others going through the same journey.

TIPS FOR OTHERS

Scoliosis and wearing a corset have been challenging in my life, but they have also provided opportunities for growth and learning. Through this experience, I have learned to value my health and well-being, accept my condition, and seek the emotional support I need. I have also developed qualities such as compassion and empathy towards others facing difficulties.

If I could give advice to those going through a similar situation, I would encourage them to seek emotional support from the beginning. Openly talking to friends, family, or seeking support groups can help alleviate the feeling of isolation and provide the necessary support to face the challenges. Additionally, try to accept your condition and do not be ashamed of it. Remember that your condition does not define you as a person, and there are many other valuable and meaningful things in life.

Focusing on small victories and learning to appreciate the things that can still be done is another important key. Despite the limitations, it is possible to find activities that bring joy and satisfaction. Furthermore, practicing self-compassion and maintaining a positive attitude can make a significant difference in how you face the situation.

In conclusion, scoliosis, and wearing a corset have left a profound impact on my life. Through this experience, I have learned to value my health, accept my condition, and seek the necessary support. I have also developed qualities such as compassion and empathy towards others. If you are going through a similar situation, remember that you are not alone, and there are resources and support available. Maintain a positive attitude and find ways to enjoy the things you can still do. Your story and experience can inspire and help others going through the same journey.

SHARE MY HISTORY

I decided to write this book because I want to help others who may be going through the same experience as me. I know how terrifying it can be to face a medical condition and feel like you're alone in your struggle. Furthermore, I want others to know that they are not alone and that there are ways to overcome the challenges that arise.

Another reason why I decided to write this book is to challenge the stereotypes surrounding scoliosis and wearing a corset. Often, scoliosis is associated with a negative image of individuals with spinal deformities who must wear restrictive devices. However, my experience proves that this is not necessarily true. I want others to realize that scoliosis is just a part of who we are, and it doesn't define our identity or our ability to live a fulfilling life.

I also want to offer a voice of hope and optimism to those facing a similar situation. Scoliosis and wearing a corset may seem like an insurmountable obstacle, but with time and determination, they can be overcome. I hope that my story provides them with the inspiration and encouragement they need to keep moving forward.

Lastly, I decided to write this book as a way to continue challenging scoliosis in my own life. I am currently fifteen years old, and soon I will have my brace removed and evaluate the possibility of surgery or not, so I wanted to somehow remember this stage for the rest of my life. Writing about my experience has also allowed me to process my own emotions and reflect on how I have grown and evolved as a person. I hope that by sharing my story, I can find a sense of closure and liberation in the future.

In summary, I decided to write this book to offer hope, inspiration, and a positive perspective to those who are going through a similar situation as mine. I hope that my story provides them with the strength and encouragement they need to overcome the challenges they face and find happiness and fulfillment in their own lives. Sharing my story has been a healing process for me, and I hope it has a positive impact on others going through a similar situation.